NAVIGATING SQUAMOUS CELL CARCINOMA WITH CONFIDENCE AND CARE

Empowering Strategies And Finding Strength For Confronting Cell Cancer For Holistic Recovery And Emotional Well-Being

DR. WESLEY IAN

DISCLAIMER

The information in this book is not meant to replace professional medical advice, diagnosis, or treatment; rather, it is meant mainly for general informational reasons. If you have any questions about a medical problem, you should always consult your doctor or another trained health expert. Don't ever discount expert medical advice or put off getting it because of something you've read in this book.

Any negative effects or repercussions arising from the usage of the material provided herein are not the responsibility of the book's author or publisher. It should be noted by readers that the material in this book is not all-inclusive and might not address every facet of the subject. Furthermore, new research may have an impact on how health concerns are understood or treated because medical knowledge is always changing.

No particular test, treatment, method, or product mentioned in this book is endorsed or promoted by the author or publisher. The reader assumes all risk associated with using the information included in this book.

Before making any big decisions regarding your health, it's crucial to speak with a licensed healthcare provider. The relationship between a patient and their healthcare practitioner should not be replaced by this book, nor is it meant to offer medical advice.

The opinions presented in this book are the author's and may not necessarily represent those of the publisher. Any errors, omissions, or inaccuracies in the information in this book are not the responsibility of the author or publisher.

It is recommended that readers independently confirm any information contained in this book and speak with a healthcare provider about their specific medical needs and state of health.

TABLE OF CONTENTS

ABOUT THE BOOK

The book "Navigating Squamous Cell Carcinoma with Confidence and Care" is a thorough resource that covers the complex terrain of squamous cell carcinoma (SCC) and offers priceless information to patients, caregivers, and medical professionals.

The book is methodically organized to provide readers with a thorough understanding of SCC, covering everything from the different forms and developmental processes to its basic concepts. The book in-depth examination of diagnostic techniques enables people to make well-informed decisions and take an active role in their healthcare process.

Most importantly, the book dives into treatment alternatives, providing a detailed rundown of strategies including immunotherapy, targeted therapy, radiation therapy, chemotherapy, and surgery. The dynamic character of medical developments in SCC management is reflected in the inclusion of developing therapeutic options.

A sympathetic examination of living with SCC is provided, which also covers coping mechanisms, emotional health, and the realities of modifying one's lifestyle both during and after treatment.

Beyond the medical realm, the guide explores the complexities of navigating the healthcare system, stressing the significance of choosing a qualified healthcare team and having successful communication. Prevention is the main focus. Readers are guided through lifestyle modifications, sun protection, and routine self-examinations to proactively defend against SCC. Long-term care and survivability are discussed, encouraging a comprehensive approach to post-treatment health.

A priceless tool, it offers a list of patient advocacy groups, online forums, support groups, and other resources so that people can connect with a strong support system. The goal and target readership of the book are emphasized in the introduction, which also provides a road map for individuals looking for support and assurance during their SCC journey. "Navigating Squamous Cell Carcinoma with

CHAPTER ONE

INTRODUCTION TO SQUAMOUS CELL CARCINOMA

THE KNOWLEDGE OF SQUAMOUS CELL CARCINOMA

One notable and common type of skin cancer that results from aberrant squamous cell proliferation is called squamous cell carcinoma (SCC). This kind of carcinoma is mainly linked to mucous membranes and the epidermis, the skin's outermost layer. To put it simply, SCC starts in squamous cells, which are thin, flat cells that resemble fish scales. It also tends to appear in parts of the body that are exposed to UV light, like the face, ears, neck, lips, and backs of hands.

DEFINITION AND FOUNDATIONS

Fundamentally, squamous cell carcinoma is a serious health concern because it can spread to other areas of the body and can infiltrate adjacent tissues. SCC is typically found in areas of the skin that have been injured by radiation, chemicals, or chronic inflammation, or where the skin has been exposed to the sun for an extended period. To better understand the condition and put into practice efficient preventive measures, it is imperative to identify the critical factors that lead to the development of SCC.

REASONS AND DANGER ELEMENTS

There are several different causes and risk factors for squamous cell carcinoma. Long-term exposure to UV radiation from the sun or man-made sources, like tanning beds, is thought to be the main cause. People who have light-colored eyes, light-colored hair, and fair complexion are typically more vulnerable to the damaging effects of UV radiation. Furthermore, disorders like actinic keratosis, which is the consequence of cumulative UV damage or a history of chronic skin irritation may increase the likelihood of developing SCC. A compromised immune system, exposure to specific chemicals and poisons, and a history of radiation therapy are additional risk factors.

VARIOUS SQUAMOUS CELL CARCINOMA TYPES

Squamous cell carcinoma manifests itself in a variety of ways, with different subtypes displaying unique characteristics. While mucosal SCC can form in the mucous membranes of organs such as the mouth, throat, esophagus, and genital areas, cutaneous SCC mostly affects the skin. Comprehending these distinct categories is crucial for precise diagnosis and customized therapeutic strategies. A biopsy is frequently used in the diagnosis process, in which a tiny sample of the afflicted tissue is inspected under a microscope to check for the presence of malignant cells.

THE DEVELOPMENT OF SQUAMOUS CELL CARCINOMA

Genetic mutations and modifications within squamous cells are part of the complex process that leads to the development of Squamous Cell Carcinoma. One of the main triggers that damage these cells' DNA is exposure to UV light. Consequently, unchecked proliferation and tumor formation result from the disruption of the regular regulatory processes that govern cell growth and division. The dynamic evolution of SCC involves the conversion of healthy cells into malignant ones, which can spread to distant organs and infiltrate neighboring tissues.

To sum up, a thorough understanding of squamous cell carcinoma necessitates knowledge of its definition, fundamentals, causes, risk factors, many forms, and the complex process of its development. This information is critical for prevention as well as early detection, highlighting the need for sun protection, routine skin checks, and timely medical intervention to lessen the effects of this common type of skin cancer.

Making a Squamous Cell Carcinoma diagnosis

Squamous cells are the thin, flat cells that are present on the skin's surface. Squamous cell carcinoma (SCC) is a kind of skin cancer that starts in these cells. Early diagnosis and treatment of SCC are essential for a better prognosis and course of treatment. A key component of treating this type of skin cancer is being aware of the symptoms and signs, the value of screening and early detection, and the necessary diagnostic tests and procedures.

Signs and Symptoms: Both individuals and medical professionals can recognize the visible signs and symptoms that are frequently associated with squamous cell carcinoma. These could include the emergence of raised, scaly growths on the skin that resemble warts or open sores and are persistent. These growths usually have an uneven border and may bleed or create crusts. SCC may also be indicated by modifications to the moles' or skin lesions' size, color, or texture. Additionally, the affected area of SCC may experience pain, itching, or tenderness. To detect these symptoms early and take appropriate action, one must be aware of them.

Screening and Early Detection: Regular skin inspections, including self-examinations by individuals and expert evaluations by dermatologists, are necessary for screening for squamous cell carcinoma. Regular skin examinations make it possible to see any worrisome growths or alterations to preexisting lesions. Fair-skinned people, those with compromised immune systems, and those with a history of extended sun exposure may be more vulnerable and should be especially watchful of their skin. Early detection is essential to stopping the spread of SCC, thus people are urged to notify their healthcare professional as soon as they see any worrying changes.

Diagnostic Tests and Procedures: When squamous cell carcinoma is suspected or found, medical practitioners use a range of diagnostic tests and procedures to confirm the diagnosis and determine the cancer's extent. Typically, a biopsy is carried out, which entails taking a tiny sample of tissue for investigation in a lab from the suspected area. This biopsy gives information about the features of the tumor and aids in determining the presence of malignant cells. Furthermore, imaging tests like magnetic resonance imaging (MRI) or computed tomography (CT) scans may be carried out to assess the cancer's extent, particularly if there is a worry that it has spread to neighboring tissues or lymph nodes.

Interpreting Diagnostic Results: Determining the meaning of diagnostic results necessitates a meticulous examination of data gathered from imaging investigations and biopsies. Under a microscope, pathologists examine the tissue samples to look for aberrant squamous cells, evaluate how differentiated they are, and ascertain the tumor's grade. The findings aid in classifying the cancer as invasive—penetrating deeper layers of the skin or spreading to other parts of the body—or in situ, meaning it is limited to the top layer of skin. Treatment planning requires an understanding of the stage and grade of squamous cell carcinoma since these factors affect the selection of therapeutic measures, such as radiation therapy, surgical excision, or topical medicines.

A thorough strategy is required for the diagnosis of squamous cell carcinoma. This includes identifying the disease's signs and symptoms, carrying out routine screening procedures, running diagnostic tests, and correctly interpreting the findings. Improving outcomes and reducing the negative effects of this prevalent kind of skin cancer on patients' general health and well-being requires prompt identification and adequate management.

CHAPTER TWO

OPTIONS FOR TREATMENT

SYNOPSIS OF THERAPEUTIC STRATEGIES

There are many different treatment modalities available for different medical diseases, and these modalities are customized to meet the individual needs of each patient. The nature and stage of the ailment, the patient's general health, and the likelihood of success in reaching therapeutic objectives all play a role in the treatment plan selection. Several treatment modalities, such as surgery, excision, Mohs surgery, and radiation therapy, will be covered in detail in this overview.

OPERATION

A common and essential therapeutic option in many medical specialties is surgery. It entails the surgical removal of afflicted organs or tissues to treat diseases like tumors, anomalies, or wounds. Reducing or eliminating the disease load, managing symptoms, and regaining normal physiological function are the main objectives of surgical procedures. Depending on the disease, surgeons use a range of methods, such as excision and specialist operations like Mohs surgery.

ELIMINATION

Excision is a surgical technique in which a margin of surrounding healthy tissue is removed together with aberrant or diseased tissue. Skin lesions, malignancies, and other localized anomalies are commonly treated with this method. The danger of recurrence is decreased by the accuracy of excision, which helps guarantee total elimination of the afflicted region. Scalpels and lasers are two examples of the instruments that surgeons may use, depending on the condition that needs to be treated and its location.

MOHS SURGERY

Mohs surgery is a sophisticated and precise surgical method that is largely used in the treatment of skin malignancies, particularly those that have a high recurrence risk or are located in cosmetically sensitive locations. The procedure bears the name of its originator, Dr. Frederic Mohs. In contrast to standard excision, Mohs surgery involves the methodical removal of tiny tissue layers, with each layer being immediately examined under a microscope. This iterative procedure minimizes the removal of healthy tissue and maximizes cosmetic results until no malignant cells are found.

RADIATION TREATMENT

Known by another name, radiotherapy, radiation therapy is a non-invasive therapeutic approach that targets aberrant cells and either destroys them or stops their growth. Although not limited to cancer, it is frequently utilized in the treatment of non-cancerous ailments.

External beam radiation is one way that radiation therapy can be administered externally. Another method is internal brachytherapy, which involves placing a radioactive source in or close to the affected area. The kind of ailment, where it is located, and the patient's general health all play a role in the radiation therapy decision.

The summary of therapeutic modalities emphasizes the significance of a customized, interdisciplinary approach to patient care. Radiation therapy offers a non-invasive option for identifying and eliminating diseased cells, whereas surgical procedures such as excision and Mohs surgery are essential for removing aberrant tissues. To guarantee the greatest potential outcome for each unique patient, choosing a particular treatment modality is a difficult decision involving coordination among healthcare specialists.

CHEMOTHERAPY

Chemotherapy, which uses medications to either kill or stop the growth of cancer cells, is still the mainstay of treatment for several cancers. Systemic administration of the medications enables them to target quickly dividing normal cells as well as malignant ones throughout the body. Chemotherapy is a successful treatment, but because it affects healthy cells, it frequently has adverse effects. These include nausea, hair loss, and decreased immunity.

Chemotherapy is being improved to be more selective to lessen the harm it does to normal cells.

IMMUNOTHERAPY

Using the body's immune system to identify and destroy cancer cells, immunotherapy is a cutting-edge method of treating cancer. Immune checkpoint inhibitors, adoptive cell transfer, and therapeutic vaccinations fall under this type of treatment. Immunotherapy aims to prevent cancer cells from using their evasion mechanisms by modifying immune responses. Even though immunotherapy has demonstrated amazing results in some malignancies, its efficacy varies, and scientists are still looking for ways to maximize and broaden its use in treating other cancer types.

PERSONALIZED TREATMENT

Drugs that explicitly target molecular changes or pathways essential for cancer cell survival and proliferation are used in targeted therapy. Targeted therapy, as opposed to chemotherapy, attempts to minimize harm to healthy cells by interfering with particular molecules involved in the cancer process. This method, which enables individualized and accurate treatment plans, is predicated on a thorough understanding of the genetic and molecular features of the malignancy. Numerous malignancies have shown benefit from targeted therapy, and continuing research involves finding new targets and improving those that already exist.

NEW APPROACHES TO TREATMENT

The frontier of cancer research is represented by emerging therapy alternatives, which include innovative approaches and treatments that exhibit potential in preclinical and early clinical investigations. Gene therapies, treatments based on nanotechnology, and creative medication delivery methods are a few of these approaches. Gene therapies seek to replace or repair damaged genes, and nanotechnology uses nanoparticles to deliver drugs specifically to specific areas of the body, improving treatment selectivity. Emerging therapies aim to overcome the shortcomings and difficulties of established treatments, opening the door for less invasive and more potent interventions.

There is constant work to increase the effectiveness and lessen the adverse effects of current treatment modalities, making the landscape of cancer treatment dynamic. Targeted therapy, immunotherapy, and chemotherapy have all become indispensable instruments in the oncologist's toolbox, each having special advantages and disadvantages. In the meantime, the investigation of novel therapeutic approaches highlights the scientific community's dedication to expanding understanding and offering more individualized and potent treatments to cancer patients.

CHAPTER THREE

COPING WITH CANCER OF THE SQUAMOUS CELLS

MANAGING THE PROGNOSIS

Being told you have Squamous Cell Carcinoma (SCC) can be a very upsetting experience emotionally. Understanding the nature of the ailment, looking into treatment possibilities, and accepting the impact on one's life are all important aspects of coping with a diagnosis. People with SCC must educate themselves about the condition, how it progresses, and available treatment options. With this information, they can be more equipped to make decisions regarding their healthcare path.

PUTTING TOGETHER A SUPPORT NETWORK

Developing a strong support network is essential to managing Squamous Cell Carcinoma. In addition to enlisting the help of medical specialists, this entails building a network of friends and family and potentially joining support organizations. The difficulties brought on by SCC can be lessened by the practical and emotional help that a support system offers. Making connections with people who have experienced comparable diagnoses can provide insightful conversations, motivation, and a feeling of belonging that enhances a person's general well-being.

EMOTIONAL HEALTH

A person's overall quality of life is significantly impacted by their emotional health if they have squamous cell carcinoma. It's important to acknowledge and communicate any emotions, including fear, sadness, and uncertainty, to manage the emotional components of the diagnosis. Getting professional counseling or therapy can help with coping strategy development and offer a secure environment for talking about feelings. A more resilient emotional state is also facilitated by joy-bringing activities, an optimistic outlook, and the maintenance of relationships in the face of SCC's problems.

CHANGING ONE'S WAY OF LIVING

Living with Squamous Cell Carcinoma frequently requires major lifestyle adjustments to support general health and treatment. Making healthier dietary choices, getting regular exercise, and giving up bad habits like smoking are a few examples of these adjustments. A new lifestyle change is frequently a slow process that calls for tolerance and flexibility. Incorporating these modifications can benefit SCC management as well as an individual's sense of empowerment and control over their health.

Receiving a Squamous Cell Carcinoma diagnosis is a difficult journey that calls for changes to one's lifestyle, support networks, coping strategies, and emotional stability. By adopting a holistic strategy that tackles the psychological, social, and physical facets of managing SCC, people can overcome obstacles more skillfully and improve their general standard of living.

Living with squamous cell carcinoma requires a multidimensional strategy that takes into account many facets of health and wellbeing, such as diet and nutrition, physical activity and exercise, and managing side effects from treatment. These elements are essential for maintaining general health, supporting the course of treatment, and improving the quality of life for those with squamous cell carcinoma.

NUTRITION & DIET

People with squamous cell carcinoma must maintain a healthy, well-balanced diet. Sufficient nourishment is crucial for bolstering the immune system, elevating vitality, and expediting the recuperative procedure. Patients are frequently instructed to concentrate on eating a diet high in whole grains, fruits, vegetables, and lean meats. Foods high in antioxidants, such as leafy greens and berries, may be especially helpful in reducing oxidative stress and enhancing cellular health. Patients must collaborate closely with healthcare providers, including dietitians, to customize their diets to individual requirements and handle any dietary limitations or difficulties that may occur during treatment.

EXERCISE AND PHYSICAL ACTIVITY

People with squamous cell carcinoma must include regular exercise and physical activity in their daily routine. Exercise has the potential to enhance general strength, elevate mood, and reduce weariness which is frequently linked to cancer and its therapies. While the kind and level of exercise may differ based on personal circumstances, walking, mild yoga, and swimming are frequently advised. Making regular exercise a priority not only improves physical health but also gives people a feeling of empowerment and control when things are hard.

HANDLING SIDE EFFECTS OF TREATMENT

Squamous cell carcinoma treatment can have a range of side effects, from minor to severe. It is imperative to efficiently handle these adverse effects to improve the general quality of life for patients receiving treatment. Medication management, lifestyle changes, and the use of complementary therapies like massage or acupuncture are some strategies for handling side effects. Self-care techniques combined with medical interventions can help manage common side effects such as nausea, exhaustion, and skin sensitivities. Having open lines of communication with medical professionals is essential to quickly identifying and resolving any treatment-related issues.

Living with squamous cell carcinoma requires a multifaceted approach that includes lifestyle modifications that promote general well-being in addition to medical treatments. Through good management of side effects from treatment, exercise, and nutrition, people can take an active role in their care, build resilience, and enhance their overall quality of life while they navigate the path through cancer.

CHAPTER FOUR

GETTING AROUND THE HEALTHCARE SYSTEM

SELECTING A MEDICAL GROUP

Making the proper healthcare team selection is essential to successfully navigate the healthcare system. Finding medical specialists who not only have the required training but also share your values and interests is the first step in the process.

Think about things like experience, credentials, and communication style when selecting a specialist or main care physician. It's critical to believe that your healthcare staff is looking out for your best interests and to feel at ease openly sharing your health issues. Making educated judgments regarding the people who will be handling your medical treatment can be facilitated by doing your homework and getting recommendations from reliable sources.

INTERACTING WITH YOUR MEDICAL TEAM

A healthy patient-doctor relationship and overall healthcare experience are largely dependent on effective communication. You may accurately convey your symptoms, concerns, and medical history when you communicate openly and honestly. To guarantee that you fully comprehend your diagnosis, available treatments, and any possible side effects, it's critical that you actively communicate with your healthcare team by asking questions and seeking clarification. Making a note of your symptoms, prescriptions, and inquiries can make your appointments more fruitful. Furthermore, by communicating any preferences or worries you may have regarding your treatment plan, your medical staff will be able to customize their care to meet your individual needs.

SECOND OPINIONS

When making healthcare decisions, getting a second opinion is a wise move. It can provide you with a new perspective on your medical situation and more information about your diagnosis and available treatments. Seeking second opinions is a proactive measure to make sure you have looked into all of the options for treatment and information. It is not a sign of mistrust. It is good to let your primary healthcare practitioner know that you want to seek a second opinion, as they can often offer insightful advice and possibly help streamline the process. Being fully informed about your medical condition gives you the ability to make decisions about your health that are well-informed.

FINANCIAL AND INSURANCE CONSIDERATIONS

Part of navigating the healthcare system knows what your insurance covers and how to handle money matters. Learn the details of your insurance policy, such as coverage limits, deductibles, and co-pays. You can use this information to make wise financial decisions about medical services and treatments. When dealing with significant out-of-pocket costs, talk to healthcare providers about payment arrangements or opportunities for financial support. Furthermore, proactively checking for and challenging billing irregularities might assist avoid needless financial hardship. Examining potential resources, including patient advocacy organizations or government assistance programs, can offer more assistance in handling the financial facets of healthcare.

CHAPTER FIVE

HOW TO AVOID SQUAMOUS CELL CANCER

SUNSCREEN AND SKIN CARE

Squamous cell carcinoma (SCC) is a form of skin cancer that develops from the squamous cells in the epidermis. It can be prevented in large part by wearing sunscreen and taking good care of your skin. Extended sun exposure is one of the main risk factors for the development of solar cortical cancer (SCC).

The damaging effects of UV radiation on the skin can be considerably decreased by utilizing sun protection techniques including wearing protective clothes, finding shade during the hottest parts of the day, and applying broad-spectrum sunscreen with a high SPF. Applying sunscreen to the face, neck, hands, and any other exposed skin is highly important. You should also reapply it every two hours, or more frequently if you perspire or swim.

Furthermore, one of the most important things in preventing SCC is to make sure you follow a thorough skin care regimen every day. This entails utilizing products with antioxidants to combat the damaging effects of free radicals on the skin, hydrating to maintain skin hydration, and gently cleaning to remove debris and impurities. Maintaining good skincare habits protects the skin from outside elements that could hasten the development of skin cancer in addition to improving the general health of the skin.

MODIFICATIONS TO LIFESTYLE FOR PREVENTION

A substantial portion of squamous cell carcinoma can be prevented by implementing specific lifestyle modifications. Giving up smoking is a crucial lifestyle change because smoking has been associated with a higher risk of SCC and other skin cancers. Smokers must prioritize quitting as part of their skin cancer prevention approach because smoking not only exposes the skin to dangerous carcinogens but also impairs the body's capacity to heal damaged cells.

Another important modification in lifestyle is to continue eating a nutritious diet high in fruits, vegetables, and antioxidants. Vibrant fruits and vegetables are rich in antioxidants, which help shield skin cells from oxidative stress brought on by outside influences. Maintaining skin suppleness and supporting the body's natural detoxification processes are two further benefits of adequate hydration for optimal skin health.

FREQUENT SKIN EXAMINATIONS AND CHECK-UPS

Frequent skin inspections and screenings are essential for identifying any skin cancers, particularly squamous cell carcinoma, early on. People should get to know their skin and keep an eye out for any changes in the moles, freckles, or other skin lesions' size, shape, color, or texture. Seeking a quick evaluation from a dermatologist is recommended for any newly developed skin growth.

Regular expert skin examinations are equally important, particularly for those with a family history of skin cancer, a history of severe sun exposure, or other risk factors. Dermatologists are skilled in spotting questionable lesions that self-examinations could miss. Early detection raises the likelihood of a successful outcome and enables prompt action.

IDENTIFYING WARNING SIGNS EARLY

It is critical to recognize the early indicators of squamous cell carcinoma to receive timely medical treatment and intervention. While there are many ways that SCC can emerge, frequent symptoms include red, scaly areas that persist, open sores that do not heal, and changes in the way that preexisting moles or skin lesions seem. To rule out the possibility of skin cancer, any unexplained changes in the skin should be checked by a dermatologist.

People should exercise extra caution when it comes to skin regions like the hands, ears, neck, and face that are frequently exposed to the sun. Self-checking regularly and being aware of the warning signs enable people to be proactive and seek medical attention as soon as any irregularities are noticed.

A comprehensive strategy that includes sun protection, good skin care, lifestyle modifications, routine skin examinations, and the identification of early warning indicators is necessary to prevent squamous cell carcinoma. Through the implementation of these measures in their daily lives, people can both lower their chance of getting squamous cell carcinoma and improve the general health and appearance of their skin.

CHAPTER SIX

LIFE AFTER AN EXTENDED MEDICAL CARE

KEEPING AN EYE OUT FOR RECURRENCE

Long-term care and survivorship require taking a holistic approach to the health of those who have finished their cancer treatment. Monitoring for recurrence is an essential part of this procedure and is a critical step in the management of patients after therapy.

To identify any early warning indicators of cancer recurrence, enable timely intervention, and improve the likelihood of effective treatment, routine check-ups and screenings are crucial. A variety of diagnostic tests, imaging scans, and physical examinations customized to the particular cancer type and the patient's medical history may be part of these monitoring efforts.

AFTERCARE

For cancer survivors, follow-up care is essential to maintaining their health and quality of life. Regular visits to medical specialists who specialize in survival are part of this continuous care, which addresses the psychological as well as the physical components of recovery. These visits help control and relieve treatment-related side effects in addition to keeping an eye out for any possible recurrence. Together with survivors, healthcare professionals create individualized follow-up programs that consider each patient's unique health requirements as well as any possible long-term repercussions of cancer therapy.

FOLLOWING TREATMENT, EMOTIONAL AND PHYSICAL WELL-BEING

One complex dimension of survivorship is one's physical and mental well-being following therapy. Many people deal with a variety of emotions as they adjust to life after cancer, such as fear, anxiety, and sadness. Support services including counseling, support groups, and mental health resources are essential in helping people deal with the psychological effects of their cancer journey. It is imperative to attend to the emotional well-being of survivors. Furthermore, survivors frequently struggle with bodily issues like weariness, pain, and shifting body image. Specialized care and rehabilitation programs can help improve physical health and encourage total recovery.

CREATING A LIFE AFTER TREATMENT

Creating a life after cancer treatment entails adjusting to a "new normal". There are several aspects to this process, such as rethinking priorities, realistic goal-setting, and routines. Plans for survivorship care may include recommendations for dietary changes, regular exercise, stress management, and other lifestyle adjustments. In the post-treatment phase, social support is especially important since survivors can often gain by relating to others who have gone through similar circumstances. Developing resiliency and discovering meaning outside of cancer treatment are essential elements of creating a happy and meaningful life after treatment.

Long-term care and survivorship go beyond the end of cancer treatment and emphasize overall health. A holistic strategy for supporting cancer survivors in their journey towards a satisfying and healthy future includes interrelated components such as follow-up care, developing a post-treatment life, treating mental and physical health, and monitoring for recurrence.

CHAPTER SEVEN
MATERIALS AND ASSISTANCE
ORGANIZATIONS FOR PATIENT ADVOCACY

Patient advocacy organizations are essential to the healthcare system because they fight for patients' rights and welfare. Usually non-profit organizations, strive to empower people with health issues by providing resources, information, and support. Patient advocacy groups support better healthcare laws, funding for research, and raising public awareness. They frequently concentrate on particular medical disorders. These groups help to create a healthcare system that is more patient-centric by elevating the voices of patients.

INTERNET-BASED COMMUNITIES

Online communities have developed into essential resources for those looking for support, connections, and knowledge about a range of health-related topics. These online forums encourage candid conversations among people with comparable experiences, fostering a feeling of empathy and camaraderie. People have a rare opportunity to share information about symptoms, treatments, and coping mechanisms in online health forums. Online health communities offer a helpful support system, but it's crucial to approach them critically and make sure the material is accurate and compliant with medical regulations.

SUPPORT TEAMS

Support groups provide a more individualized and personalized kind of help for people dealing with health issues. Support groups, whether they convene in person or digitally, unite people who can relate to one another's hardships. Leaders of these groups could be medical professionals or people who have firsthand knowledge of the illness. Support groups enhance emotional support, lessen feelings of loneliness, and promote camaraderie via sharing shared experiences. When it comes to managing chronic conditions, support groups can be especially helpful as they assist people in navigating both the practical and emotional parts of their health journey.

FURTHER READING AND SOURCES

For those who want in-depth information on particular medical illnesses, therapies, and procedures, Additional Reading and References are crucial components. People can get a lot of information from books, articles, research papers, and reliable websites to help them make decisions about their health.

Furthermore, reading more can enable a person to actively participate in conversations with medical experts, which promotes shared decision-making. Reliable sources guarantee that people have access to reliable and evidence-based information to improve their understanding of health-related topics. Examples of these sources include peer-reviewed publications and recognized medical institutes.

Resources and support in the healthcare field cover a wide range of approaches, each with a special function in empowering people individually and collectively.

Patient Advocacy Organizations, Online Communities, Support Groups, and Additional Reading and References work together to create a comprehensive network of care that helps people navigate the complex world of healthcare by promoting mental wellness, knowledge, and awareness.